LIFESTYLE HABITS

FOR
LASTING POSITIVITY

JACKI DASLIMER
PRESTON MITCHUM JR.

ISBN: 978-1-956581-57-7

ERIN GO BRAGH
Publishing
Canyon Lake, Texas
www.ErinGoBraghPublishing.com

TABLE OF CONTENTS

INTRODUCTION

"WITH HOPES THAT
THIS BOOK INSPIRES JOY
AND CONFIDENCE WITHIN YOU
AS YOU TAKE THIS
POSITIVE JOURNEY TOWARDS
A BETTER, HEALTHIER YOU!"

PRESTON MITCHUM JR

INTRODUCTION

In this journey we call life, cultivating the right mindset and habits is fundamental to building a healthy, positive lifestyle.

Health coach Jacki Dalsimer and "Mr. Positivity" Preston Mitchum come together to share insights on how to nurture balance and positivity within ourselves, providing the foundation for lasting transformation.

This book offers practical advice and powerful, inspirational insights designed to help you achieve your goals and build the life you envision.

From cultivating a resilient mindset to fueling our bodies with what they truly need, each element contributes to creating the best version of ourselves.

By developing these positive habits and incorporating the power of affirming words, we lay the groundwork for a balanced, fulfilling life.

Our mind, body, and soul each require nourishment—powerful, uplifting influences that ignite our inner superpower.

Together, let's explore how we can inspire, uplift, and empower ourselves to become the best possible versions of who we are, sharing that light with the world.

LIFESTYLE HABITS FOR LASTING POSITIVITY

PAUSE AND LET THESE WORDS INSPIRE YOUR NEXT STEP

Pause. Be still. Allow your mind, body, and soul to align with the endless possibilities of what your future can become. Within these pages, you'll discover words designed to uplift and empower, inspiring you to embrace a lifestyle of health, positivity, and purpose.

Take this moment to let your spirit absorb the positive energy already flowing within you—an energy that will be magnified by the affirmations and encouragement awaiting you here. Let this be your reminder that you are capable of becoming the very best version of yourself, one step, one thought, and one moment at a time.

POSITIVE THOUGHTS. POSITIVE VIBES

WEIGHT
MANAGEMENT

WEIGHT MANAGEMENT

You glance in the mirror and feel a desire for change—a vision of a healthier, more fit version of yourself that you know would boost your confidence and energy. But the journey seems overwhelming, as weight management has been a challenge for you in the past.

The journey begins with mindset.

Embracing real, lasting change requires a shift in perspective. You need to be ready to commit to a healthier lifestyle to create the version of yourself you envision.

From there, it is all about building a foundation of supportive habits, and that's where I, Coach Jacki, come in.

As your health coach, I'm here to guide you toward sustainable weight management through nutrition, movement, and mindset practices that align with your goals.

One of the biggest shifts is moving away from the idea of "losing weight" as the ultimate goal. Instead, it's about embracing a lifestyle of balance and wellness.

Think of it as a way of treating your body with kindness and respect—nourishing it with the right foods, hydrating regularly, and finding joy in movement.

This isn't about deprivation or rigid diets; it's about creating a life where you feel good, both physically and mentally.

Daily actions build a foundation.

Start with simple steps, like focusing on nutrient-rich meals and taking time to truly savor what you eat.

Hydration is essential too, as water supports every system in your body and helps regulate hunger.

Physical activity doesn't have to be a chore; it could be as simple as a brisk walk, dancing, or a short strength workout, anything that keeps you moving and feeling energized.

Evenings are a time to reset.

Wrap up your day with a calming ritual: a bit of meditation, a few deep breaths, or a moment to reflect on positive affirmations.

This not only helps quiet the mind but it also helps prepare your body for quality sleep, which is an often-overlooked aspect of weight management.

Achieving your weight goals takes a mix of strategies, a blend of nutrition, exercise, sleep, mindfulness, and self-compassion.

When all these elements come together, you're not just managing your weight; you're shaping a lifestyle that can bring you lasting change and fulfillment.

Over time, these habits will become part of you, creating a healthy rhythm that you can carry with you for years to come.

DAILY HABITS

In this chapter, we will explore essential habits that can significantly enhance your overall health and well-being.

By focusing on these practices, you can improve your physical and mental state while also achieving long-term sustainable wellness.

The following key points highlight some of the most impactful habits for a healthier lifestyle:

1. **Mindful Eating:**
   Take time to eat slowly and savor each bite to improve digestion and avoid overeating.

2. **Regular Hydration:**

Aim to drink at least 8 cups of water per day to help control hunger and support metabolism.

3. **Consistent Exercise:**

Incorporate at least 30 minutes of physical activity daily, mixing cardio and strength training.

4. **Balanced Meals:**

Plan meals with a balance of protein, healthy fats, fiber, and complex carbs to stay full longer.

5. **Adequate Sleep:**

Aim for 7–8 hours of quality sleep, as poor sleep can disrupt hunger-regulating hormones.

CHALLENGES

Overcoming daily challenges related to health and fitness requires small but intentional steps. Here are some strategies to help you tackle common obstacles and stay on track:

1. Managing Cravings:

Combat cravings by focusing on nutrient-dense low glycemic meals* based around a lean protein. Steer clear of sugar and low fiber carbohydrates.

*Nutrient-dense, low-glycemic meals are those that provide a lot of essential nutrients, such as vitamins, minerals, fiber, and protein, without causing a spike in blood sugar levels.

2. Finding Time for Exercise:

Fit in short exercise sessions throughout the day, even if it's a quick walk.

3. Avoiding Processed Foods:

Reduce reliance on processed foods by meal-prepping with whole ingredients. Avoid the inner aisles of the grocery store.

4. Social Settings:

Navigate social events by choosing healthier options and practicing portion control. Remember it is ok to politely say no.

5. Stress Management:

Practice stress-reducing activities, like short meditations throughout the day, since stress can lead to overeating.

A LITTLE POSITIVITY TO CARRY YOU THROUGH THE DAY.

We all come in different shapes and sizes, and achieving and maintaining a healthy weight can be challenging. One of the first steps is to set personal weight goals that feel right for you.

There's no expectation for us all to look or feel the same. What matters is finding what feels healthy and sustainable for you. When you reach that point, you'll feel the positive impact on your life. With a balance of nutrition, exercise, supportive people, and stress management, these elements work together not only to help you reach your weight goals but also to support the positive, evolving person you are becoming.

POSITIVE THOUGHTS, POSITIVE VIBES

HYDRATION

THE IMPORTANCE
OF HYDRATION

We've all heard the phrase: drink enough water. Hydration isn't just a health tip; it's essential for a balanced, vibrant lifestyle.

With the hustle and bustle of daily life, it's easy to overlook the importance of staying hydrated, but the benefits are undeniable.

As a health coach, I can't stress enough the importance of drinking enough water each day. Carry a water bottle with you, add natural flavors like lemon or cucumber if needed, and make a conscious effort to skip sugary drinks.

Sugary beverages not only add empty calories, but they also contribute to health issues like high blood pressure, diabetes, and high cholesterol.

Consider this: according to research, up to 75% of Americans are chronically dehydrated, which can lead to fatigue, headaches, poor concentration, and even mood swings.

Water makes up about 60% of the human body, and every cell, tissue, and organ depend on it to function properly. Staying hydrated can boost your energy, improve digestion, and aid in maintaining a healthy weight.

Creating a hydration habit can be simple. Start by adding a glass of water to every meal, or set small reminders throughout the day to take a sip. With consistent hydration, you'll likely notice positive changes in your skin, improved sleep, and better physical movement.

Remember, a well-hydrated body is a healthy body. Embracing this small habit can have a big impact on your overall well-being, helping you thrive physically and mentally every day.

DAILY HABITS
FOR STAYING HYDRATED

Making hydration a part of your daily routine can help you stay energized and healthy. Here are some simple habits to incorporate into your day for consistent hydration:

1. **Start with Water:**

    Begin your day by drinking a glass of water as soon as you wake up to kickstart hydration after a night's rest.

2. **Carry a Water Bottle:**

    Keep a reusable water bottle with you throughout the day, so it's always accessible.

3. Set a Hydration Schedule:

Aim to drink water at specific times, like before each meal, mid-morning, and mid-afternoon. This creates a routine that makes hydration automatic.

4. Add Flavor if Needed:

Use natural flavor enhancers like lemon, cucumber, or mint to make water more enjoyable, especially if you find plain water bland.

5. Eat Water-Rich Foods:

Include hydrating foods like cucumbers, oranges, watermelon, and soups in your diet to boost hydration.

6. Use Reminders:

Set a phone alarm or use an app as a reminder to drink water, especially if you tend to get busy and forget.

7. Track Your Intake:

Keep a mental or written note of how many cups or ounces of water you've had each day to make sure you're meeting your goal.

SMALL CHALLENGES
FOR HYDRATION

Staying properly hydrated is key to maintaining energy and overall health. Here are some small hydration challenges to help you stay on track throughout the day:

1. **Try an Extra Glass Per Meal:**

   Challenge yourself to drink an extra glass of water with each meal to increase your daily intake.

2. **Replace One Sugary Drink:**

   Swap one soda, juice, or other sugary drink with water to encourage healthier hydration.

3. Hydration Test:

Check your urine color periodically–light yellow generally indicates good hydration. Try to keep it at this level throughout the day.

4. Finish a Bottle by Lunch:

Challenge yourself to drink a full water bottle by midday. This prevents you from needing to drink too much late in the day.

5. Hydrate Before and After Exercise:

Make it a habit to drink water before you start working out and again afterward, as your body loses fluids when you sweat.

CARRY THIS MESSAGE WITH YOU AS A BEACON OF LIGHT

(Along with a bottle of water.)

Yes, I get it—you're always on the go, juggling responsibilities, and sometimes hydration slips through the cracks.

But remember, nourishing your body with the essentials, especially water, is one of the simplest yet most powerful ways to support your mind, body, and spirit.

Hydration is foundational to a balanced, vibrant life. When you make drinking water a daily habit, you'll feel its positive impact—from increased energy and mental clarity to a greater sense of well-being.

Embrace hydration as a gift that you can give yourself, one sip at a time, every single day.

POSITIVE THOUGHTS, POSITIVE VIBES

NUTRITION

NECESSARY NUTRITION

You've likely heard the saying, "You are what you eat." Nutrition truly is the foundation of our health and vitality.

The foods we put into our bodies fuel us, helping us perform at our best—mentally, physically, and emotionally. Nourishing ourselves with the right balance of nutrients is essential to creating a vibrant, energized life.

For a well-rounded diet, aim to incorporate fresh fruits, lean proteins, healthy fats, and complex carbohydrates into your meals. Health coaches everywhere emphasize the importance of these core elements.

Small, balanced meals throughout the day, with snacks rich in nutrients, lean proteins, and fresh vegetables, can keep your energy steady and your mind sharp.

Of course, we all know how tempting those donuts, burgers, fries, and cookies can be. While they might be delicious, processed foods like these don't provide the nutrients our bodies need for sustained energy and wellness.

Regular indulgence in high-sugar, high-fat foods has been linked to weight gain, heart disease, and other health issues.

Balance is key. Treat yourself every now and then, but make nutrient-dense foods the cornerstone of your diet.

Taking time to eat mindfully—like chewing thoroughly and savoring each bite—also helps with digestion and prevents overeating.

Don't stress if it feels challenging at first. Create a simple meal schedule or system that works for you, making it easier to incorporate nutritious foods consistently.

Start small, maybe by swapping one snack a day with a healthy option or adding an extra serving of vegetables to dinner.

Remember, every small change counts. By fueling yourself with the right nutrients, you're setting yourself up for a healthier, happier life.

DAILY HABITS
FOR BETTER NUTRITION

1. Eat Breakfast Daily:

Start with a balanced breakfast that includes protein, healthy fats, and complex carbs to fuel your morning.

2. Plan Meals in Advance:

Spend a few minutes planning meals or snacks for the day to avoid unhealthy last-minute choices.

3. Add More Fruits and Veggies:

Aim to include at least one serving of fruits or vegetables in every meal for added vitamins and fiber.

4. Choose Whole Foods:

Opt for whole, unprocessed foods (like whole grains, lean proteins, and fresh produce) whenever possible.

5. Practice Mindful Eating:

Focus on eating without distractions, paying attention to hunger and fullness cues to prevent overeating.

6. Include Healthy Snacks:

Keep healthy snacks like nuts, yogurt, or fruit on hand to avoid reaching for less nutritious options.

7. Drink Water Before Meals:

Having a glass of water before meals can help with digestion and prevent overeating by keeping you hydrated.

SMALL CHALLENGES FOR BETTER NUTRITION

Improving nutrition can be achieved through small, manageable changes that make a big impact over time. Here are some simple challenges to help you develop healthier eating habits:

1. **Go Meatless Once a Week:**

   Try a vegetarian or plant-based meal at least once a week to explore more plant-based options and improve nutrient diversity.

2. **Add One New Vegetable:**

   Challenge yourself to try a new vegetable each week to add variety and explore different nutrients.

3. **Reduce Sugary Foods:**

Pick one day each week to reduce added sugars by avoiding sugary snacks, drinks, or desserts.

4. **Choose Whole Grains:**

Replace refined grains (like white rice or bread) with whole-grain options (like brown rice, quinoa, or whole wheat) to increase fiber intake.

5. **Eat Slowly and Chew Well:**

Make an effort to chew food thoroughly and eat slowly to enhance digestion and help you feel full.

FUEL YOUR SPIRIT WITH THIS UPLIFTING REMINDER.

Yes, I was once that person, hitting the gym every day, feeling like I was putting in the hard work but not seeing the results I wanted. The missing piece was nutrition—fueling my body with the right foods and staying hydrated. A balanced combination of nutrition and exercise is essential to reaching our full potential.

Surrounding ourselves with positive, supportive people can shape the mindset we need to create that balance and become the best versions of ourselves.

POSITIVE THOUGHTS. POSITIVE VIBES

STRESS MANAGEMENT

STRESS MANAGEMENT

Waking up with gratitude is one of the best ways to start the day on a positive note and minimize stress. While stress is a natural part of life, our ability to manage it greatly influences the positive lifestyle we want to create.

As a health coach, I share key strategies with my clients to help them reduce stress not only throughout the day but also in challenging situations.

One essential practice is learning how to say "no." Avoiding the temptation to overload yourself with commitments can significantly reduce stress. This creates space for balance and helps you focus on what truly matters.

Developing relaxing techniques is also crucial. Find methods that work for you, whether it's deep breathing, meditation, or a short walk in nature. These small, intentional moments of peace help recharge you, giving you the mental clarity to handle daily tasks with ease.

Getting a good night's sleep and prioritizing nutrition are equally important. Quality sleep allows your body and mind to recover, while nourishing foods support a relaxed and focused mindset. Both are foundational to stress management.

Identifying specific stressors in your life and either eliminating or minimizing them is also key. As health coaches, we experience stress too, and managing it effectively is a daily practice.

By identifying and addressing our stress points, we build resilience.

Incorporating these daily habits, along with pinpointing the challenges in your environment that might be adding to your stress, are vital steps toward a lifestyle filled with positivity and peace.

DAILY HABITS
FOR STRESS MANAGEMENT

The following will aid you in developing good daily habits to help control your stress and manage your positivity.

1. **Morning Breathing Exercise:**

   Start the day with 5–10 minutes of deep breathing or meditation. This sets a calm tone for the day and improves focus.

2. **Set Intentional Breaks:**

   Schedule short breaks during your day to step away, stretch, or take a walk. These breaks help clear your mind and recharge your energy level.

3. Limit Screen Time:

Try to limit non-essential screen time, especially before bed, to help improve sleep and reduce anxiety.

4. Healthy Eating:

Eat balanced meals throughout the day and avoid skipping meals. Eating consistently helps maintain energy levels and reduces irritability.

5. Express Gratitude:

Write down 1–3 things you're grateful for each day. Focusing on the positive aspects of life can improve mood and reduce stress.

6. Stay Active:

Incorporate some physical activity, even if it's just a brisk walk. Physical movement releases endorphins, the body's natural stress relievers.

7. Journaling or Self-Reflection:

Spend a few minutes each day journaling or reflecting. This can help you process emotions and gain clarity on stressful situations.

SMALL CHALLENGES FOR STRESS MANAGEMENT

Managing stress can be a series of small adjustments that make a big difference. Here are a few simple strategies to help you reduce stress and promote a sense of calm in your daily life:

1. Try a New Relaxation Technique:

Experiment with yoga, progressive muscle relaxation, or guided imagery to find a relaxation method that resonates with you.

2. Practice Saying No:

Challenge yourself to decline one non-essential obligation to make room for relaxation and self-care.

41

3. **Reduce Caffeine Intake:**

Try lowering caffeine by switching to herbal teas or water to help reduce anxiety and improve sleep quality.

4. **Set a Digital Detox Goal:**

Pick one day a week to reduce social media usage or spend the evening without screens, allowing more time for offline relaxation.

5. **Add a Positive Affirmation:**

Start each day with a positive affirmation, especially one related to handling stress, like "I can handle whatever comes my way today."

ALLOW THIS THOUGHT TO BRIGHTEN YOUR PERSPECTIVE.

Stress is a word we all know too well. Life can feel overwhelming, with long lists of tasks each day and never enough time. So how do we manage stress? This is something most of us search for daily. Many would say that creating a positive balance is the key.

Start by setting an intentional tone for your day, prioritizing what truly needs your energy, and identifying and minimizing sources of stress. Equally important is creating safe spaces where we can talk openly and find support. None of us has all the answers, but together, we can foster an environment that helps us find balance and move toward where we want to be.

POSITIVE THOUGHTS. POSITIVE VIBES

EXERCISE

EXERCISE IS JUST MOVEMENT

Many of us may not fully realize the importance of daily movement and exercise for overall health. Yet, incorporating regular activity into your routine is crucial—not only for keeping your muscles strong and your joints flexible but also for supporting mental well-being and energy levels.

Building an exercise routine that includes daily movement is a powerful step toward a healthier lifestyle. When you set specific goals, you're laying the groundwork for progress. These goals give you purpose and help break down the journey into manageable steps, making it easier to stay on track. As a health coach, I'm here to support you not only with a nutrition plan but with a customized exercise regimen designed to help you feel strong, energized, and confident.

It's natural to look at images on TV or in magazines and admire the fit, muscular physiques we often see. But remember, those results didn't happen overnight—it's a marathon, not a sprint. Adopting that same mindset will allow you to appreciate each small victory along the way, embracing gradual progress rather than chasing quick fixes.

A strong support system can make all the difference in keeping up your motivation. Surround yourself with like-minded individuals who are committed to feeling and looking their best.

Whether through a workout group, a fitness class, or a personal trainer, being part of a supportive environment fosters accountability and encouragement when you need it most.

We all have those days when motivation feels low, when the thought of hitting the gym seems like a big hurdle. Trust me—I've been there too! But the benefits of consistency are immense, both physically and mentally.

Integrating exercise as a regular part of your life becomes something you'll depend on, a non-negotiable element of your healthy lifestyle. Embracing this commitment will help you cultivate lasting well-being, strength, and confidence—allowing you to thrive for years to come.

DAILY HABITS

Building positive daily habits can help make exercise a consistent part of your routine. Here are some simple strategies to incorporate physical activity into your day and stay on track:

1. **Set Small, Attainable Goals:**

   Aim for short-term, achievable workout goals (e.g., 10 minutes of stretching or a quick walk) to build consistency.

2. **Exercise at the Same Time Each Day:**

   Establish a routine time for exercise, whether morning or evening, to build a steady habit. Schedule your work-outs like doctor appointments.

3. Mix Up Workouts:

Be sure to incorporate strength, cardio, and flexibility exercises to keep things interesting and improve overall fitness.

4. Track Progress:

Keep a simple log of exercises, reps, or minutes completed to stay motivated and see improvements over time.

5. Warm Up and Cool Down:

Prepare your body with a 5–10-minute warm-up and end with a cool-down stretch to reduce injury risk.

CHALLENGES

Staying consistent with exercise can be challenging for many reasons. Here are some common obstacles and tips for overcoming them to maintain a regular fitness routine:

1. **Finding Motivation:**

   Staying motivated daily can be tough. Try setting a reminder or pairing exercise with a favorite activity, like listening to music or a podcast.

2. **Time Constraints:**

   A busy schedule can make it hard to fit in workouts. Break exercise into smaller chunks, like 5–10-minute intervals throughout the day.

3. **Boredom with Routine:**

Doing the same workouts can feel monotonous. Consider trying new activities like cycling, yoga, or HIIT to keep things fresh. Find a group fitness class or a workout buddy.

4. **Overcoming Plateaus:**

Hitting a plateau can be frustrating. To progress, adjust your routine with new exercises, higher intensity, or added weights.

5. **Managing Soreness and Fatigue:**

Exercise can lead to muscle soreness. Prioritize rest days and use foam rolling or light stretching to aid recovery.

START YOUR DAY WITH AN EMPOWERING THOUGHT.

Daily movement is essential for building a positive and healthy lifestyle. Whether it's a walk, a run, or a strength session at the gym, working our muscles and keeping our bodies flexible makes a big difference.

For those with desk jobs, it can be incredibly challenging to stay active, but taking time during lunch breaks or right after work for a hike, jog, or bike ride can be just what we need to get energized.

Keep moving, and you'll definitely feel the boost in your energy!

POSITIVE THOUGHTS. POSITIVE VIBES

SLEEP

THE IMPORTANCE OF SLEEP

It's a common refrain: sleep just isn't your friend. As a health coach, I hear this almost daily from clients who feel defeated by restless nights and groggy mornings. So, how do we achieve that elusive good night's sleep?

The answer is different for each person, influenced by lifestyle, stress, and personal circumstances. But one thing is certain: quality sleep is foundational, setting the tone for a balanced and productive day.

Mr. Positivity himself, Preston Mitchum, often encourages sprinkling positive, peaceful practices into our daily routine— a kind of spiritual seasoning that helps us find calm in the midst of life's noise.

The path to restful sleep often begins with examining our lifestyle. Prioritizing what truly matters, and recognizing what can wait, is an essential step in creating balance. When we avoid overloading our minds and bodies, we allow space for tranquility to flourish.

Proper nutrition also plays a vital role; a well-rounded, nourishing diet supports our body's natural rhythms, making it easier to drift into restorative sleep.

Personally, I've found that surrounding myself with peace-promoting activities like walking, hiking, meditation, and connecting with people who radiate the kind of energy I seek has transformed my approach to rest. These daily practices build a foundation of calm that I can carry with me into the night, encouraging my body to relax and welcome sleep naturally.

Health coaching has given me a unique perspective on sleep challenges. Every client's journey is distinct, shaped by individual habits, dreams, and obstacles. Yet, despite these differences, a common thread unites us all—a desire for true rest, for the renewal only deep, peaceful sleep can bring.

In the pages that follow, I'll outline some of the most common sleep challenges people face and share daily habits that can help you on your journey to better rest. With intentional shifts in our daily routine, we can invite tranquility into our lives and create the conditions for a more restful, fulfilling night's sleep.

COMMON SLEEP CHALLENGES

Many people struggle with falling or staying asleep due to a variety of factors. Here are some common sleep challenges that can interfere with getting a restful night's sleep:

1. **Stress and Overthinking:**

   Difficulty shutting off racing thoughts or worrying about the day's events.

2. **Inconsistent Sleep Schedule:**

   Irregular bedtimes and wake-up times disrupt the body's internal clock.

3. Heavy Meals, Caffeine or Alcohol Close to Bedtime:

Eating large meals or consuming caffeine late into the evening can hinder relaxation and prevent sleep.

4. Screen Time Before Bed:

Exposure to screens (phones, computers, TVs) emit a blue light, which can interfere with melatonin production. Aim for a digital sunset at least an hour before bedtime.

5. Lack of Physical Activity:

Insufficient movement during the day can make it harder to wind down at night.

DAILY HABITS
FOR BETTER SLEEP

1. Establish a Relaxing Bedtime Routine:

Wind down with calming activities like reading, gentle stretching, or deep breathing exercises.

2. Maintain a Consistent Sleep Schedule:

Go to bed and wake up at the same times every day, even on weekends, to strengthen your internal clock.

3. **Limit Alcohol, Caffeine and Heavy Meals in the Evening:**

Try to avoid caffeine after midday. Limit your alcohol consumption. Eat lighter dinners to support relaxation before you go to bed.

4. **Create for yourself a Comfortable Sleep Environment:**

Keep your bedroom cool, dark, and quiet, and invest in a quality mattress and pillows.

5. **Incorporate Daily Movement:**

Aim for regular exercise, like a morning walk or evening yoga, to help reduce stress and improve sleep quality.

BREATHE IN, FOCUS, AND EMBRACE THIS MESSAGE.

We all know the importance of sleep and the impact it has on our day. Yet, many of us struggle to get the quality rest we need.

By nourishing our bodies with balanced nutrition, staying active, and surrounding ourselves with positive, supportive people, we can improve the quality of our sleep and, in turn, our energy and focus.

A restful night allows us to be our most productive, vibrant selves, radiating the positivity the world needs. Embrace the value of a good night's sleep, and commit to small habits that help you get there.

POSITIVE THOUGHTS, POSITIVE VIBES

MENTAL WELLNESS

MENTAL WELLNESS

Building mental wellness is a journey that unfolds gradually, often through the power of small, consistent habits. Over time, these habits accumulate, fostering a deeper transformation in your mental state and overall well-being.

On this Positive Vibes movement, I emphasize that mental wellness practices aren't just tasks to check off a list— they're fundamental to living the lifestyle you envision for yourself.

Gratitude lies at the heart of mental wellness. When we cultivate gratitude, we learn to appreciate the present moment and value what we have. Take a few moments each day to reflect on the blessings in your life. This isn't just about acknowledging what's good; it's about shifting your perspective to find positivity, even in challenges.

Visualizing what you want to achieve while remaining grounded in what you already have creates a powerful balance, helping you stay motivated yet content.

Good mental health often begins with how we nourish our bodies. When we eat well, our bodies feel good, and in turn, our minds follow.

Nutrition isn't just about fueling physical energy; it's a cornerstone of mental clarity and resilience. By consistently choosing foods that support a healthy body, we create a foundation for mental well-being that enhances our focus, mood, and overall outlook on life. This is why I emphasize a lifestyle approach over temporary diets; it's about creating a sustainable way of eating that supports both body and mind.

Daily affirmations and meditation are simple yet powerful practices that build mental resilience and positivity.

Affirmations reinforce self-belief, helping you stay aligned with your goals and values, while meditation grounds you, providing a space to breathe, reflect, and reset. Together, these practices foster a stable mindset that can better weather life's inevitable ups and downs.

Equally important is surrounding yourself with positive influences—people who lift you up and situations that add joy to your life. The energy of those around you can be a vital part of your mental well-being.

It's a holistic approach that encourages lifestyle changes, inspiring us to pursue being our best selves in every way.

By thinking beyond the scale and embracing a mindset of growth and self-improvement, we honor the connection between mind, body, and soul. Our bodies are temples, and to truly thrive, we need to nurture all three aspects to align with our vision of wellness.

The essentials of mental wellness often lie in the basics: moving our bodies, eating well, resting deeply, and engaging in activities that bring us joy. Regular exercise releases endorphins, which naturally elevate our mood, while a balanced diet keeps our energy stable throughout the day.

Quality sleep, too, is indispensable; a rested mind can tackle challenges with clarity and calm. Finally, make time for hobbies and moments of joy—they aren't indulgences, but vital components of a healthy mind.

Life can be demanding, especially when people around us need our help and support. It's easy to feel stretched thin, which is why setting boundaries is essential to maintaining your mental wellness. Prioritizing yourself isn't selfish; it's necessary.

By creating space for self-care, you're better able to meet both your needs and the needs of others. Balance requires intentional effort, but by respecting your own limits, you create a life that supports and sustains your mental well-being.

DAILY HABITS

1. Practice Gratitude:

Start or end each day by listing a few things you're thankful for. This helps shift focus to positive aspects of life.

2. Physical Activity:

Even a short walk or quick workout can boost endorphins, reduce stress, and improve mood.

3. Mindfulness Meditation:

Set aside 5-10 minutes for meditation or deep breathing exercises to reduce anxiety and increase focus.

4. Stay Connected:

Reach out to friends or family daily, even if it is just a quick text or call. Social connections are essential for emotional well-being.

5. Healthy Boundaries:

Protect your time and energy by setting limits on work, social media, and other stressors.

6. Sleep Hygiene:

Aim for 7-8 hours of restful sleep by setting a regular bedtime and reducing screen time before bed.

7. Balanced Nutrition:

Eating regular, balanced meals, particularly those rich in vitamins and minerals, supports both physical and mental energy.

COMMON CHALLENGES

1. Consistency:

Sticking to wellness routines can be tough, especially on busy or stressful days.

2. Negative Self-Talk:

It's easy to get caught up in self-doubt. Try to replace negative thoughts with constructive or compassionate ones.

3. Overwhelm:

Balancing daily obligations with wellness practices can sometimes feel overwhelming. Start small and build up gradually.

4. **Stigma:**

Talking openly about mental health can still feel challenging due to stigma, but finding safe spaces to discuss it can be beneficial.

5. **Comparisons:**

Social media and societal pressures can lead to unhealthy comparisons. Remember, wellness is personal, and your journey is unique.

PLANT A SEED OF ENCOURAGEMENT IN YOUR HEART TODAY.

To live the healthy and positive lifestyle we desire, everything begins with our mental wellness. It starts with nurturing our souls and awakening the positive energy within our minds. By focusing on restoring balance and harmony in our thoughts, we lay the foundation for true well-being—mind, body, and soul.

When our minds are centered and our spirits renewed, our bodies, our sacred temples, will reflect that wellness. Positive thoughts are the seeds from which positive actions grow, shaping the life we envision. Embrace this truth and let your journey to wholeness begin from within.

POSITIVE THOUGHTS, POSITIVE VIBES

POSITIVE MINDSET

POSITIVE MINDSET

Some call me Mr. Positivity, my friends call me Preston. As I reflect on my life, I'm struck by the many changes and challenges I've faced along the way. My years as a journalist at WMAR-TV Baltimore, covering stories across Maryland, taught me about the spectrum of human experience. Every night, I was immersed in the struggles, triumphs, and daily lives of our community, and it made me deeply aware of how much a positive mindset matters, no matter what life throws at us.

In 2015, my life was irrevocably changed when I lost my father to a sudden heart attack at just 67. That was one of the toughest seasons I've endured, and like so many, I turned to what comforted me most: sharing thoughts and positivity on social media. It became a form of therapy, a way to process my grief while trying to lift others. One day, my dear friend Kathleen J. Shields, who has been instrumental in publishing my Positive Vibes books, suggested something that would change the course of my work and purpose: daily affirmations.

"Preston," she said, "your words could inspire the community. Why not give people something uplifting to hold on to each day?"

That conversation stayed with me. Kathleen was right—affirmations are powerful! They can reframe our thinking, help us see the good even in hardship, and, more than anything, remind us of our strength.

Together, Jacki and I set out to create this book, hoping that these conversations, reflections, and affirmations would empower you to build a positive mindset, even on the hardest days.

Each of us leads a unique life, navigating different paths and obstacles. It's no secret that staying positive can be a struggle at times. But ask yourself this: would you like to feel more joy?

Do you have a sense of what steps you can take to cultivate a more fulfilling, optimistic life? What are the obstacles, past or present, that may be holding you back from a true sense of positivity and peace? These questions might seem simple, but they're powerful, and the answers are deeply personal.

For some, optimism is a conscious choice, a decision to view the world through a lens of hope and possibility. For others, it's a journey, requiring small, intentional changes and a willingness to let go of what no longer serves them. A positive mindset doesn't happen overnight, but it's within reach.

Consider the people around you: Are they the voices that uplift, inspire, and challenge you to grow? Or are they voices that drain, discourage, or instill doubt? Sometimes, a more positive mindset begins with a reevaluation of our surroundings and relationships, as well as our thoughts and habits.

Now is the time to be kind to yourself, to grant yourself grace as you journey through the challenges and triumphs of life.

This is also the perfect time to take a close look at what your life looks like today. What minor changes can you make that will move you closer to a mindset rooted in positivity, gratitude, and resilience?

Every chapter in this book is designed to guide you, step by step, toward the mindset you seek. Give yourself permission to start this journey, and remember that small shifts—whether in thoughts, habits, or the people we surround ourselves with—can lead to transformative changes.

A positive mindset isn't about avoiding life's challenges; it's about facing them with courage, optimism, and the belief that brighter days are always ahead.

DAILY HABITS

1. Morning Affirmations:

Start each day by speaking or writing a positive affirmation: *"I am capable of handling today's challenges."*

2. Gratitude Practice:

Write down 3 things you're grateful for each day, focusing on both big and small aspects of life.

3. Mindful Breathing or Meditation:

Spend 5–10 minutes each morning or evening focusing on your breath to clear your mind and center yourself.

4. Acts of Kindness:

Do one kind thing for someone daily, whether it's a compliment, a small favor, or a simple thank-you note.

5. Physical Activity:

Move your body daily with a walk, stretch, or workout to boost endorphins and release tension.

6. Positive Consumption:

Limit negative media and instead engage with positive content like inspiring books, podcasts, or music.

DAILY CHALLENGES

1. Reframe Negative Thoughts:

Whenever a negative thought arises, challenge yourself to reframe it with a positive angle. For instance, replace "I'm not good enough" with "I'm doing my best and growing every day."

2. Limit Complaints:

Try going a full day without complaining. Instead, focus on solutions or ways to make peace with minor inconveniences.

3. Self-Reflection:

At the end of the day, reflect on one positive thing you did, said, or experienced.

4. Say No to Self-Criticism:

Catch yourself when you're being overly critical and replace it with self-compassionate language.

5. Stretch Outside Comfort Zone:

Each day, try one small thing that feels challenging or new to build confidence and resilience.

TAKE A MOMENT TO REFLECT ON THIS TRUTH.

You've likely heard it time and time again: positivity is the key. And it's true—a positive mindset is essential for creating balance and attracting the uplifting energy we want in our lives. However, cultivating this mindset requires intention and effort.

It begins with the choices we make each day. Surround yourself with uplifting people who inspire and support you. Fill your mind with encouraging thoughts, read daily affirmations, and seek out words that motivate and empower you. Each of these practices contributes to building the positive mindset you need to thrive and create the life you envision. Remember, positivity isn't just something you stumble upon; it's a mindset you nurture and grow.

POSITIVE THOUGHTS, POSITIVE VIBES

CONCLUSION
& ACTION
PLAN

Staying Consistent with Nutrition:

Knowing what foods truly nourish our bodies can be challenging, especially with so many processed options available.

Consistency in choosing wholesome, nutrient-rich foods over convenience items can feel difficult to maintain.

Understanding Food's Role and Impact:

Sometimes, we struggle to understand what "healthy" food really is and what a balanced meal looks like. This confusion can lead to trial and error, making it hard to find a sustainable routine.

Managing Daily Stress:

Balancing daily tasks while minimizing stress takes intentional planning.

Prioritizing what matters and letting go of non-essential tasks can feel overwhelming, especially without clear boundaries.

Cultivating a Supportive Social Circle:

Surrounding ourselves with positive, uplifting people is crucial, but it's often hard to find and maintain relationships that inspire and support our growth.

Recognizing who lifts us up and who may drain our energy can be a process.

Building Daily Growth Habits:

Creating daily routines that help us grow into the people we aspire to be requires dedication. Habits take time to develop, and it can be hard to keep going, especially when results don't appear immediately.

Staying Consistent with Exercise:

Moving our bodies regularly is essential, yet maintaining this consistency is often a challenge. Busy schedules, fatigue, or even lack of motivation can disrupt exercise routines, making it tough to establish a lasting habit.

Struggling with Snacking and Sugar Cravings:

Many of us face cravings for snacks and sugary treats that can feel difficult to control. Reducing these habits requires discipline and self-awareness, as well as understanding the reasons behind our cravings.

Taking That First Step Forward:

Knowing we're not content with where we currently are is one thing, but finding the courage to take that first step toward change can feel daunting. Trusting the journey and leaping forward, even with uncertainty, is often one of the greatest challenges.

The Importance of Accepting and Loving Ourselves as We Are:

Looking in the mirror and embracing who we are in each stage of growth can be hard. Self-acceptance requires a grace and patience as we strive to become the best versions of ourselves.

LET THIS AFFIRMATION GUIDE YOUR JOURNEY

The inspirational words and insights from this book are your tools to craft the positive action plan you need to embrace a healthy, fulfilling, and uplifting lifestyle. By integrating this empowering knowledge into your daily life, you will foster the harmony your mind, body, and soul require to thrive and become the best version of yourself.

Creating this plan is only the beginning. Surround yourself with people who uplift and support your vision—those who will help you stay focused and see it through. Taking this step forward is not just necessary; it's transformative. Your journey toward balance, positivity, and purpose starts here.

POSITIVE THOUGHTS, POSITIVE VIBES

ABOUT PRESTON

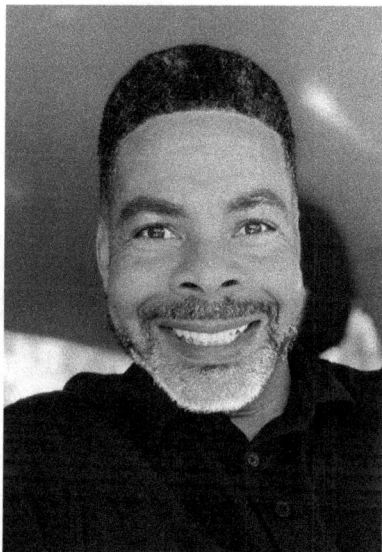

Preston Mitchum Jr. has dedicated his life to giving back and making a difference. Born in Bronx, New York his family moved to Langley Park, MD in 1981.

His family established the Mitchum Lawn and Landscaping business shortly after. Preston's father, Mitchum Sr. worked here for over 30 years, creating beautiful lawns and establishing relationships throughout the community.

Preston Jr. is a graduate of Towson State University where he took his love for video and became an 18-year veteran news photographer for WMAR-TV in Baltimore, Maryland.

During this time, he founded The PMJ Foundation to create change in the Baltimore community. The foundation's vision is to impact families through programs and services that offer positive growth. The foundation has served thousands throughout Maryland.

With the passing of his father, Preston has taken over the family business and will continue to provide the quality service that his family established for many years.

THE PMJ FOUNDATION

Presenting Possibilities for Brighter Futures

The PMJ Foundation's Career Awareness Project (CAP) after-school program brings the outside professional world into the classroom. Community volunteers present their careers to our participants which engage our at-risk youth to explore the infinite possibilities of college and career choices that are available.

To learn more about the PMJ Foundation please visit: www.pmjfoundation.org

A portion of the proceeds of these books will support the programs that the PMJ Foundation offers.
Preston hopes that the positive message this book has to offer will impact thousands and create positive vibes that we all can feel.

OTHER BOOKS

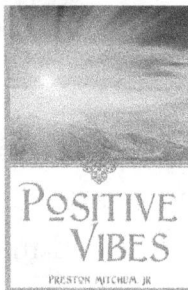

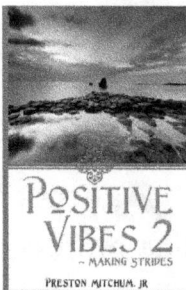

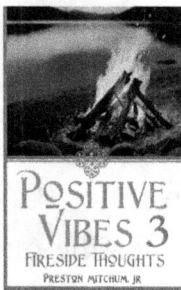

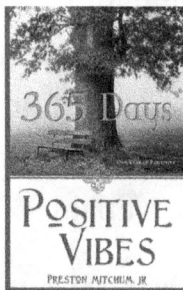

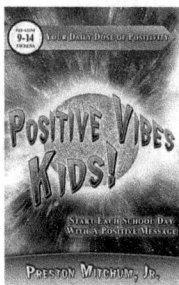

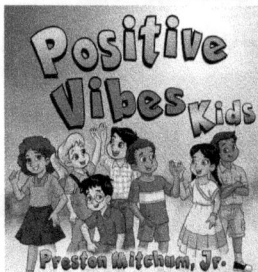

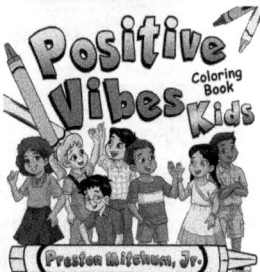

ABOUT JACKI

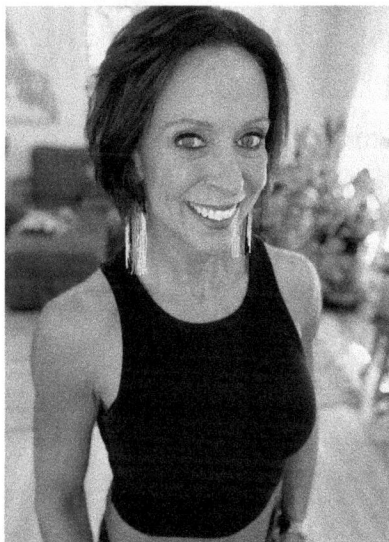

Jacki Dalsimer is a passionate health coach with a mission to inspire and guide others toward living a healthier, more vibrant life. With over 20 years of experience in the health and wellness industry, she is a firm believer that the foundation of a long, thriving life lies in the way we nourish our bodies, hydrate, move, sleep, and manage stress. Her journey into health coaching began in her early twenties after being diagnosed with thyroid cancer at the age of 20. This life-altering experience ignited a deep passion for holistic health, prompting her to explore and embrace a lifestyle that prioritizes well-being at every level.

Having faced personal health challenges and witnessed the impact of mindful living on her own recovery, Jacki became dedicated to helping others achieve lasting, sustainable health. She's seen every fad and quick-fix approach come and go, but one truth has remained clear: without establishing solid, healthy habits, nothing

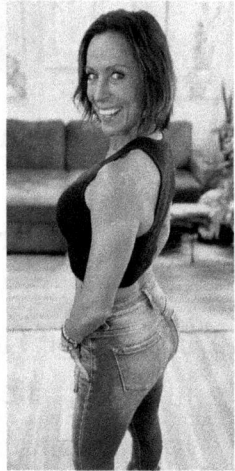

works in the long term.

With a deep commitment to empowering individuals to make positive, lasting changes, Jacki brings a wealth of knowledge, personal experience, and compassion to her work. Through her coaching, she strives to help people create a balanced, resilient life—one that fosters not only longevity but a high quality of life that can be enjoyed at any age.

Jacki's philosophy is simple yet transformative: true health comes from consistent, thoughtful choices in how we care for ourselves. And by nurturing our bodies in a holistic, sustainable way, we unlock the potential for a healthier, longer, and more fulfilling life.

ERIN GO BRAGH
Publishing

Erin Go Bragh Publishing publishes various genres of books for numerous authors. Their portfolio consists of a 1200-page Vietnamese to English Dictionary, Historical fiction, an award-winning children's educational series, multiple adult novels and memoirs, tween adventure stories, as well as Christian Fiction. Their objective is to promote literacy and education through reading and writing.

www.ErinGoBraghPublishing.com
Canyon Lake, Texas